Medicine

History of Medicine: The Most Important People and Discoveries Through The Ages Including: Alternative Medicine, Remedies, Nursing, Modern Cancer Treatments, & Anti Aging

reliable complete information. No warranties of any kind are expressed or implied. Readers acknowledge that the author is not engaging in the rendering of legal, financial, medical or professional advice.

By reading this document, the reader agrees that under no circumstances are we responsible for any losses, direct or indirect, which are incurred as a result of the use of information contained within this document, including, but not limited to, —errors, omissions, or inaccuracies.

Table of Contents

Introduction

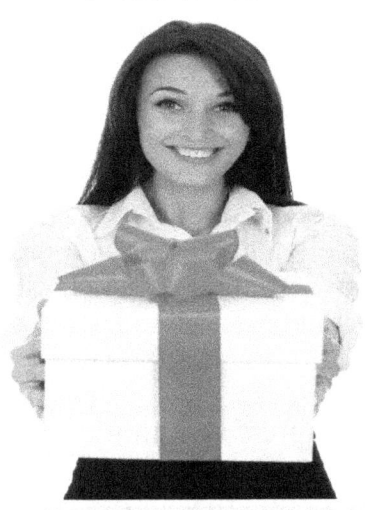

The history of medicine traces far back in history to the point where techniques to heal a person came around the same time as the first tools ever created. People would always work to find research to increase the medical field and be able to find more information to help the health of the society surrounding them. They worked to understand a multitude of different techniques to find the symptoms of every disease they encountered and were exposed to.

From the first tools came the experience of surgery. From a man named Hippocrates came the origin from the 'Father of Medicine. From the cellular research of biology came the reasoning behind how viruses developed. All of these things together created the medical system known today in our own modern age.

In this collection of chapters and information surrounding the history of medicine, it is all a quick summary to show how it all came to be. An introduction to your own personal research. With history, information always continues with how things came to develop and how things came to become part of the world.

Medicine is not just a hard faculty. It is a lifetime of studying; it is life. You have to love your job in order to be a good doctor. You have to be ready to get up in the middle of the night from your warm bed and to save someone's life. You have to be ready to miss some beautiful events in your life in order to serve your job. If you are not ready for tears, back pain, blood and sleepless nights, you cannot be a physician. But as soon as you save someone's life, you will realize that it was absolutely worth everything. It was worth all the suffering, no social life, neck pain, back pain, muscle atrophy, missed events, missed opportunities, under eye bags and other not such pleasant things that come with being a doctor. This job is one of the greatest things in the world; not everyone can do it, and not everyone can handle everything that comes with it. It is not just the blood. You have probably heard that you cannot become a doctor if you are afraid of blood – that is a myth. Of course, there will be blood but there any many fields of medicine where doctors do not even see the patients, especially not their blood. If you think you have the potential to change the face of medicine, to change the world and save lives – you should become a doctor. Do not let your fear and insecurities to keep you away from the greatest job that humanity has ever seen. Do not let your bad thoughts to influence the way you think about saving lives. Many doctors say that they would not do it again if they could. They would not choose medicine or go to medical school. Do not learn from them if your dream is to be the healer, the helper, and the saver. Some people say that doctors are the extended hand of God. They are probably right. Doctors do not get to choose whether they can save someone and certainly they cannot save everyone. But they try, they really do. It is actually the greatest and the worst job in the same time. Medicine does not only involve doctors. It involves nurses and other very important people who are the part of the medical team. Every one of them has their role in the system, and they have their game. Without the nurses and technicians who work so hard – doctors could not do their job as good as they do it with the help of the medical team. Nobody likes the doctors (except those who are married to them) and visit the doctor's office might seem like the worst thing that you have to do. Behind the office doors, there is a person who has spent all her/his life studying to help you and other people like you. Do you feel any better now? It would be insane to study medicine for money – anyone who is a medical student would tell you it is absolutely not worth it. Medical students (most of them) do not do it for the fame; they do not study because someone told them do (some of them do, but very few continues after the first year) and they do not do it for respect. They do it because they love to help people, they love to serve humanity and save lives. Some say that the enthusiasm goes away after the first few years, but it is not the case in every med student's life. Some of them truly and deeply believe that they can make the world a better place. And some of them succeed to do so.

Chapter 1: Hippocrates

In medical history, Hippocrates was a Greek doctor who is sometimes seen as the father of modern medicine. He was born on the Greek island called Kos (around 460 BC). His formal name was Hippocrates Asclepiades, meaning descendant of Asclepius. Asclepius was a Greek god of medicine in Greek mythology.

He was able to find fame with the other Greek doctors as he wrote a collection of medical books that created the 'Hippocratic Oath' for doctors today. 'Hippocratic Oath' is an oath which delivers the message: Do no harm. Doctors must take an oath before they start working as medical professionals. Ludwig Edelstein translated the original version of the Hippocratic Oath and the modern version of it was created in 1964 by Louis Lasagna. Louis Lasagna was a physician and a professor of medicine. "Lasagna's Oath" is accepted by many medical professionals and institutions worldwide.

Hippocrates claimed that diseases were triggered when there is something wrong in the body. Also, he believed that all diseases had a specific reason why they occur. He and some of the other Greek doctors thought that the work done by any doctor should be kept separate from the work done by another priest. They also started to observe patients more carefully. They thought that the observation of every individual patient was a very important aspect of medical care. While the ancient Greek doctors examined their patients, Hippocrates wanted more of a system for the respect of the patients and periods of observation. They recorded what was observed and created the 'clinical observation' of today. During these times, the Greek doctors were told to look at the patient's face. If the patient would look like their normal self, it was seen as a good sign. If they had a sharp nose, cold ears, hollow eyes, dry skin on the forehead, or a strange face color, it was seen as a bad sign and the beginning of an illness. This face also means that death is near. The body is giving up; it is weak. Usually, the first thing that you notice is concavity of cheeks. The patient with 'facies Hippocratica' soon starts to show some other symptoms that will later result in death (refusing food or drinks, irregular pulse, and heartbeat, skin turns purplish or gray, gasping, no urination, no bowel movements, etc.) He also described Hippocratic fingers, more known today as nail clubbing or digital clubbing. This condition is related to many diseases, but in most cases, it is related to heart and lung problems. It can be associated with lung cancer, tuberculosis, lung abscess, cystic fibrosis, hypoxia, congenital cyanotic heart disease, malabsorption, cirrhosis, Crohn's disease, Graves' disease, etc.

He also developed ways of fixing broken bones and his researches lead to the discovery of Aspirin later on.

After the doctor examined the patient carefully, they were told to begin asking questions. They were told to ask about how much sleep the patient has been receiving if they have been eating and if they have had any kinds of pain. These doctors were trained by Hippocrates to note specific symptoms and observed what happened to the ill patients on a day to day basis. This would be able to create a natural history of any illness and therefore forecast the development of the disease in another person in the future. He and the other Greek doctors all worked with the assumptions that diseases were always a natural cause instead of a supernatural cause. Priests believed that the gods caused illnesses. Because of the two different perspectives on disease, it was important for the patient to only see one side for medical treatment in order to ensure a full and healthy recovery.

Hippocrates made a big contribution to medical practice. Some doctors forget that they heal humans and observe them as things. One of the most important things in medicine is ethics. Doctors get more information when they allow the patients to tell them what they are comfortable telling them. When that does not happen, 'by the way syndrome' occurs. It means that the patient (who did not feel comfortable saying something in front of the physician) says the most important things on his/her way out. Doctors should always listen to their patients and provide necessary care. One of Hippocrates's famous quotes says: "Wherever the art of Medicine is loved, there is also a love of Humanity." This means that the doctor must be a decent, nice human being before being a medical worker! Good doctor-patient relationships will bring much better results in treatment and provide much better care for the patient. Medicine is art. Medicine is not just simple prescription writing or lab tests reading. A patient is a person, just like the doctor, who is afraid and uncomfortable. Nobody likes to be sick or go to the doctor's office. It is in human's nature to be afraid of everything.

Hippocrates also founded a school of medicine on Kos. He has spent a lot of his time teaching, traveling and practicing medicine. His students, first of all, his sons and his son-in-law, continued his researches and his practice. They wrote 'The Hippocratic Corpus' collecting his studies. In his time, corpse dissections were strictly forbidden. He had troubles with that because Greeks had much respect for dead people and human bodies. It is believed that he would have made many more discoveries if he had the permission to find out what is inside the bodies without violating the law.

He put a special accent on good diet and exercising. He also had a theory of humors. Hippocrates believed that human body consists of 4 humors - blood, phlegm, yellow bile and black bile. Hippocrates believed that it was an imbalance between those four humors that caused sickness and that they need to be balanced all the time. This theory has been proven wrong.

Doctors after Hippocrates had better hygiene. They also had less sexual relations with their patients. Hippocratic Oath promoted that doctors must never hurt their patients intentionally and that they must not take patient's money or gifts for better treatment.

Chapter 2: Vaccines

"For just a few dollars a dose, vaccines save lives and help reduce poverty. Unlike medical treatment, they provide a lifetime of protection from deadly and debilitating disease. They are safe and effective. They cut healthcare and treatment costs, reduce the number of hospital visits, and ensure healthier children, families, and communities." – Seth Berkley, CEO of Gavi, Vaccine Alliance

Vaccines have become an important part of medicine and have worked to save many lives in the past fifty years. While medical procedures and medicines are very important, vaccines are forprevention to keep people away from a harsher form of a disease. They are helping your body to fight many types of infections. The history of how these came into existence goes all the way back to Ancient Greece and follows through the different cultures throughout the world.

The Greek historian Thucydides in 429 BC was able to see that people who received a disease were less likely to get it again. With the smallpox plague that spread in Athens, people who survived the plague did not become infected a second time with the disease. In the year 900 AD, the Chinese were able to discover and find a form of a vaccine they called variolation. The point was to prevent the spread of smallpox by exposing healthy people who have never received the illness to small tissue scabs that caused the disease in the first place. They were able to do this in two ways. The first way was that they put the tissue under the skin. The second way was by putting powdered forms of the scab tissue up their nose. These variolations spread around the world in the 1700s and arrived in England in the early 18th century. During this time, smallpox was the largest infectious disease in Europe that caused the death of one-fifth of the population. While these vaccines did cause mild illnesses in people, it rarely ended in death. This meant that the rate of people getting smallpox were lower in the places that tried getting the vaccines.

The vaccinations were growing in support as they were proved to work by the scientific community in the year 1796. As this support grew, the government began to fund the research for more vaccines that first became popular in Europe and spread over to the United States. Since these were still seen to be new, some people questioned if it would really work. They wondered if this was a scam to make a person sick. Others thought that it took away a person's civil liberties.

As the public media added controversy to these vaccines, scientists in the 1880s were still continuing to develop new forms of vaccines and began research to understand exactly how a disease worked. They studied the symptoms and how the earlier vaccines were created. Eventually, they discovered a rabies vaccine and other antitoxins for tetanus and diphtheria. This started a new research and a new age for medicine. Basically, a vaccine is a biological preparation made from weakened microbes. The microbes are inserted into the bloodstream, and your immune system destroys them. It also remembers them and the next time you are really exposed to the microbes (larger amount) – it will destroy them instantly. Vaccines have saved many people's lives. Vaccination is the most effective way to prevent infectious diseases.

American Academy of Pediatrics claims that vaccines are about 95% effective in preventing some diseases. Vaccines have saved a lot of lives, including children and old people as the most vulnerable population groups. However, vaccines have a small amount of risk – one in about a million children dies from a severe allergic reaction. Scientists think that these deaths are not related to vaccines at all. Always make sure that your child's doctor is familiar with your child's allergies. It is important for all parents to know that this small risk is not so dangerous comparing to the diseases that can be prevented with vaccines. More people die from diseases than vaccines. There will always be skeptics, but it is on you to decide whether you or your child should get vaccinated. In some countries, some vaccines are a 'must, ' and they are defined by law.

Chapter 3: Antibiotics

Antibiotics are a treatment option that works against infections that are caused by bacteria. They are a variety of substances that are created from bacterial sources or microorganisms that can control the growth of bacteria. In history, it can be separated into two groups, early history, and modern history.

In early history, it goes back to ancient times with the Greeks. The Greeks and Indians worked to use molds and other plants surrounding them to treat infections. Over in Greece and Serbia, mold bread was used to treat the infections found in people. In Russia, they used warm soil to treat people. Sumerian doctors used a beer soup mixed with snake skins and turtle shells. Babylonian doctors would heal the eyes of their patients using the mixture of sour milk and frog bile.

In modern history, England, France, and Germany were able to find more treatments. In England, John Parkington used mold for treatments, Sir John Scott Burdon-Sanderson found that culture fluid covered in mold did not produce bacteria, Joseph Lister worked with antibacterial action on human tissue to find PenicilliumGlaucium, John Tyndall furthered the research on PenicilliumGlaucium, and Sir Alexander Fleming found that enzyme lysozyme and penicillin from the fungus PenicilliumNotatum. In France, Louis Pasteur found out that bacteria could kill other bacteria, and Ernest Duchesne was able to heal infected guinea pigs from the disease typhoid by using the mold PenicilliumGlaucium. In Germany, Gerhard Domagk discovered Prontosil.

Sir Alexander Fleming was one of the main people that was able to change and define the new horizons for modern antibiotics. The discovery of penicillin was able to perfect the treatment of other bacterial infections such as tuberculosis, syphilis, and gangrene. He also was inspired to discover a natural antiseptic enzyme called lysozyme. It existed in tissues, mucus, tears, and egg white. But it did not have much of an effect on bacteria. This overall led him to the discovery of penicillin.

Penicillin is the first antibiotic in the world, and it is made from fungus. It only cures the bacterial infections. It is never used to treat virus infection. When the patient takes the antibiotic, it kills most of the bacteria. Patients should never take it without doctor's supervision. Some bacteria need time to be killed, so patient must not stop taking medicine before the doctor says so. Also, specific bacteria are affected by a certain antibiotic. However, not every type of bacteria requires the same treatment and same amount of antibiotic. Bacteria can become resistant to antibiotic, and that is one of the big problems in the process of healing.

Like any other drugs, antibiotics can give you some side effects. They can be usual like nausea, and they can sometimes be pretty bad and even lead to death. Babies, old people, chronic patients, patients with kidney problems, liver failure, pregnant women (and breastfeeding women) are at risk and need to take antibiotics very carefully. Doctors must ask for your history of using antibiotics and see whether you had some problems, allergies, respiratory and other problems. The dose is the key.

Antibiotics are not the solution for all health problems. Your immune system will probably solve some things on its own like sinusitis, cold, sore throat, cough, runny nose, etc. Actually, using antibiotics for 'virus problems' can increase the chance of becoming antibiotic resistant. Do not use someone else's

[17]

drug. It is ignorant, and you can have some serious health problems later on. Use what is prescribed to you and do not share it. It is not a candy bar. Also, do not use it the next time you get sick. Go to the doctor's office again and ask for help. Do not do anything that will harm you and make you feel even worse. Even doctors go to visit other doctors for advice. Why would not you? Keep the drugs away from children and store them in cool and dark places. Do not mix them with alcohol. Read the instructions carefully and stick to them.

Chapter 4: Age Of Enlightenment

In the Age of Enlightenment, science in medicine was able to see an age of high esteem and increased physicians that were able to upgrade their social status by becoming more scientific. The health field was becoming crowded with surgeons and charlatans.

This period began in the Glorious Evolution which was founded in 1688 in England. As a new reform movement, there was a shift in values and other social policies. There was a rejection of previous thinkers and social constraints that were able to bring a spark to the Enlightenment period. These thinkers went under the banner of natural evolution in medicine instead of hiding through the concepts of equations.

The Enlightenment was able to establish a positive view and optimistic outlook for people to follow. This allowed for the role of medicine and the benefits of health to progress in the future. A confidence in contemporary thinkers that believed that health was truly a natural state for the body to follow. It could be maintained and protected to force all diseases to eventually be eradicated.

Chapter 5: Herbal Medicine

Herbs were the oldest use of medicine to be found in history. The ancient Chinese, Egyptians, and Indians used herbal remedies by combining the plant fibers around them for physical and spiritual healing purposes. They were able to preserve the ideas of infections and they experimented with healing through the power of nature.

The ancient Greeks and Romans were both widely known herbalists. They developed surgeons that were able to travel through with the armies in the Roman empire and the colonies in England. They preserved their knowledge from the other lands around them since they believed in the personal healing powers of the spirit. They could build upon their own knowledge given to them through the reflection of the monks. By not spreading knowledge, they could have a unique culture for the gods to be directed upon.

At the same time, in an Islamic conquest of North Africa, the Arabic scholars were able to discover the medical texts from the Greeks and Romans. This led to an important ancient facet of herbalism, astrology. They connected the different herbs of the region with the different kinds of people that came for help. They would treat different parts of a person's body depending on what their zodiac sign was. The medical scholars would prescribe them an herb from the same astrological sign. This was because they believed strongly in the connection between the stars and the operations of the herbs. Healing the pain through the pre-defined nature found in space and time. A person's zodiac sign would tell a medical professional which kind of medicine the person needed without looking at their own symptoms.

Many doctors forget that herbal medicine was the start of the medicine we know today. At first, herbs were the only medicine and people have always found new ways to use some plant. The easiest thing for a doctor is to prescribe something that you can buy in the pharmacy – but it is not always the best thing to do. However, drugs are not always safe and herbs are not always the best solution.

Herbal and pharmaceutical drugs have an important role in medicine. Altogether, Americans spend ten times more money on pharmaceutical drugs (about $200 billion in a single year). Anyone who went to the doctor and got out of his/her office, have asked themselves – what should I do? What is the safest option for me? Everybody wants the best remedy, the most effective one, the less harmful one, the less expensive one, etc. There are many factors included when choosing the best solution. Generally, people tend to use herbal drugs anyway, because they believe that herbs do not have bad side effects and they cost less than pharmaceutical drugs. However, herbal drugs are not as safe as you think. Yes, they have been used for centuries, and they are the gift from Mother Nature, but that does not mean that you can use it as you like.

Chapter 6: Modern Medicine

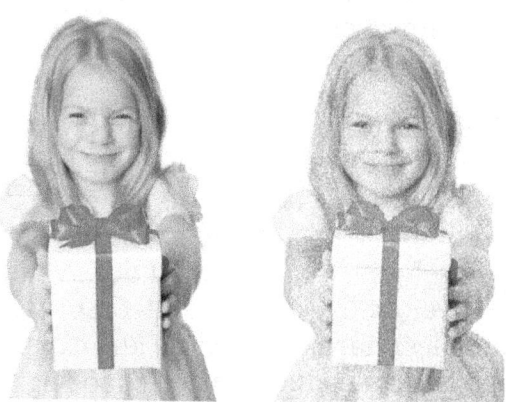
In the history of modern medicine, it is always found to be the development of disease prevention. Working to heal the sick and find new treatments for illnesses. This happened from the prehistoric times all the way to these modern times of medicine. At the beginning when unwritten history is not the easiest to interpret, scholars have been able to find that there are many cases of folklore and spiritual power to diagnose people. While times have changed in the process of healing, the respect for the patients has remained the same.

Modern medicine in the 19th century expanded quickly with the following of the increasing industry. Economic activity was able to grow rapidly with this industrial growth. The old ideas of how the infectious disease was distributed throughout the body lead to the ways of virology and bacteriology. Microbiology was then able to make its own advantages and experiment upon more microorganisms.

Cities started to grow rapidly, and doctors saw a connection between the growing population and the spread of disease. They found the diseases such as typhus and cholera to become more common. One easy way they were able to increase the health of the population was by increasing the political message of hygiene. In the years of 1818 to 1865, a doctor named Ignaz Semmelweis saw that doctors who did not wash their hands before touching the women in child labor caused the childbed fever death rates of the infants.

Since these things kept increasing, postal and communication greatly improved as well. Medical information was then able to spread faster between the scholars and medical professionals from around the world. Democracy was growing in the nation and causing people to demand health as a natural human right. Scientists advance towards disease resistance and vaccines to find more information towards illness. These few things were important towards the society of health, especially during the times of war. Technology would develop with the information to create more efficient and an easier time of innovations in surgical techniques.

Chapter 7: Obesity

Obesity has always been known to be the lack of will power and not enough exercise in a person's diet. Modern research fulfills this definition as historic research shows more of a possible connection between the genetics of people and their weight. The scientific research has gone through the scholars and philosophy of centuries to initiate the knowledge of biologic mechanisms.

For more than a century, physicians have been proposing their own ideas that obesity comes from a function of heredity. Exogenous obesity is where the food consumption of a person is more of an excess while endogenous obesity is caused more so by the hypometabolism or other thyroid disorders. These would develop from the previous generations of the person eating more food than the average and slowly forcing the future generation to adapt to a lower metabolism. For example, if an early family ate more to become obese, they could continue the trend through to the next family and cause their own children to have a natural different metabolism since the previous two families had too much energy and chemicals in their systems. While they had lots of vitamins, they also put in many fats that carry on through genetics.

In 1950, Jules Hirsch worked to show that people who were naturally obese would suffer from a lifetime struggle. Even when they would be able to shed a large amount of weight because of calorie restriction, they would still have to work with their own metabolic rates. During the calorie reduction, their metabolic rates decrease, but this causes problems on its own. For example, if a woman goes from 200 lbs to 130 lbs, she would need to consume fewer calories compared to another person that was also 130 lbs. This research led to prison feeding experiments in the 1960s. They would feed the inmates enough to increase their metabolic rates in response to their own calorie consumption. The men that had a harder time maintaining a weight gain also had a hard time shedding the weight they had. They realized that the ones with a family history of obesity supported the notion that obesity was heritable.

By 1986, the University of Pennsylvania took on their own experiment that included looking over adoption records to find people of a certain height or weight that also families of another height or weight. They used the data to compare the body mass indexes of the parents with those of the people who were adopted themselves. They were able to find that even though they had shared an environment, the adopted person's body mass index matched their own biological parents rather than those of their own adopted parents. This proved that obesity could easily be genetic rather than inherited through the surrounding environment.

At first, obesity is not a big problem if you decide to cope with it. It probably started when you looked yourself in the mirror, and you did not feel like yourself anymore. As soon as you realize that being overweight is not just the looks, you step on the right track. Being overweight is so much more.

It is related to a number of health problems that do not include zipper and skinny jeans problems. Obese people are more likely to suffer from a lot more diseases than those who are not. Obese people tend to have diabetes, heart problems, respiratory problems, troubles when walking and also get depressed and anxious. Very few people are satisfied when obese. The key lies in complete lifestyle change. It is like a makeover, but much harder.

Nowadays, many people deal with obesity. Some think it is not a problem and continue their lives with the same habits that led them to obesity. Others try to improve themselves. No one has the right to judge the ones who decide to do nothing. It is their body and their life. It is horrible when people say horrible things about people who are obese. It would certainly be good for obese people to work on their habits and eating disorders. If one decides to lose weight, he/she should start by making a plan. That plan should have an eating schedule, exercising schedule, goals (daily, monthly, year) and the person should stick to it. You should never starve yourself. It is one of the worst mistakes in this process. It is important to count the intake of calories and does enough exercise to lose them. Food gives you the energy to do everyday tasks, and it is impossible to live without basic nutrients. The body needs sugar, fats, proteins, and vitamins. If you only eat salad, you are not going to get enough energy, and you will probably end up depressed (and feeling guilty) in McDonald's in two days. Food is not the problem. You can practically eat whatever you want – as long as you watch the intake. You should eat enough not to be hungry, but know your limits. Do not be frustrated if nothing happens for a few months; every good change needs some time. It is important to believe in you and to be patient. If you stress yourself about it, it will do you harm. Stress never helps, and it will not help you to lose weight. It will probably encourage you to eat even more. Hold on to your plan and believe in yourself. Pick food that is healthy and good for your body and try to avoid food with a lot of sugar or fats. Avoid sodas, coke, chips, alcohol, white sugar, artificial sweeteners, white carbohydrates (white bread, bagels, pasta), bacon, French fries (and generally fried food), etc. It is much better to cook food instead of frying. Avoid eating out; you might think that you do not have time to prepare some food – but you know you do.

Your body wants you to take good care of it. It wants your attention and care. It is showing you that there is something wrong in what you do and that you need to fix it.

Chapter 8: Nursing

The word nurse comes from the Latin word 'nutrire'; meaning to suckle. This meant that these were the people who would care for the infirm. From the earliest times, cultures would produce a stream of nurses to follow that were dedicated to the service only on religious principles. Over in Europe, before the foundation of nurses was created, Catholic nuns and their military would provide nursing services to other people. In the 20th century, nursing then became an actual profession as an option for people to follow.

Around 100 BC, India stated that a good medical practice would require a patient, a physician, a nurse, and medicine. They believed that the nurse needed to be knowledgeable and skilled at preparing dosages of medicine to people. They also needed to be very clean people that were kind and sympathetic towards people. The nurses in this time were used as a market to bring people to health and bring people to a center that they could find medicine. They did not want people to stay home and pray for health, they wanted people to move to the nurses for medicine in order for them to collect information on diseases and the formation of illnesses.

The collection of Christian emphasis was a practical charity that would also give a rise to the development of nurses. At the end of the persecution of the churches, people in 480 AD to 547 AD began to develop more hospitals and provide more rulings towards the sympathy of giving nurses. The ancient church leaders would give the idea of medicine as an aid to hospitality. If people came to them for medicine and health, they were welcomed into a place of warmth and giving people. These nurses lived for a long time in religious communities and worked for the care to heal other illnesses.

Some of these hospitals would build up libraries and training programs within them in order to encourage people to become a part of the medical community. They were able to provide their own medical and pharmacological studies in the forms of manuscripts. When they would provide indoor medical care and allow people to stay for research in training, it developed the ideas of modern hospitals. This increase in innovation was driven by a combination of Christian mercy and Byzantine inventions. The Byzantine hospital staff themselves would include the chief physician, professional nurses, and the orderlies. Their facilities would include systematic treatment procedures and specialized research information for various diseases.

The medieval hospitals in Europe followed a rather similar pattern compared to the Byzantine medical techniques. They were all religious communities that provided nursing care through both nuns and monks. Some of these monasteries attached to the hospitals and were able to provide income for their own levels of support. Others would fund refuges for the poor or for the pilgrims. Not all of them cared for the sick as they believed in both physical and spiritual health. They wanted to increase the foundation of their own hospitals while keeping the purity of the church as a mission for Christians to follow.

Some people say that being a nurse is one of the hardest jobs in the world. Nurses have to deal with blood and other body fluids, revolting smells, infections, feces, etc. Their job is to take care of people in any conditions and any moods. Nurses touch them, help them and do not always such pleasant things. Not everyone is suitable for this job. Nurses are the 'eyes' and 'ears' of the hospital. Patients tend to vomit or urinate themselves, but nurses must remain respectful to them.

Cleaning up is not as easy as it seems. It is the living people we are talking about. Patients sometimes feel embarrassed due to their illness, but nurses have to be patient and help them. They must hide their natural reaction to smells and disgusting things. It can be awful, messy, traumatic, but it is the part of the job. Nurses deal with a lot of stress often in very bad conditions. They are great multitaskers, team workers and sometimes they take their work home. It is nothing like taking paperwork or unfinished documents. Nurses take images of their patients, questions and insecurities. Did I do it well? Did I make a mistake? Is he/she going to fine? etc. There is definitely a difference between working with computers and working with people. It is not easy when somebody trusts you, relies on you and depends on you. Nurses must never let their mood or personal issues take over. It would be a complete disaster. Patients must receive full care and proper treatment prescribed by a doctor. Nurses follow the orders and do their best to help the patients. It is not just the patient, though. Nurses must cope with entire family, relatives, friends, neighbors, work colleagues and other people that come to visit the sick person. Usually, it is hard for them to accept the fact that their loved one is sick. It is hard for practically anyone to see someone in pain and suffering. It is also hard to focus on the work when there are so many people telling the nurse that she is not doing her job right. Of course, not all nurses are angels, but most of them give their heart and soul out there to make someone more comfortable. It is not just the pillows that need to be lifted, not only food, sheets, clothes changing, bathing – it is making someone's life easier in the moments when they feel bad. Being a nurse is much more than being just a part of medical staff. She/he is a friend in distress. Some people do not even want to be comforted; not every patient is patient. Not every patient is thankful for their work. Some patients yell, scream, curse and even spit on the nurse s – and he/she needs to deal with it. No matter what race, religion, age, gender, nationality - the nurse must take care of any patient.

Chapter 9: Cancer

Cancer has been found a countless number of times through the work of many forms of research with doctors and scientists from around the world. The discoveries in anatomy, physiology, epidemiology, and chemistry created the field of oncology found today. The advances in technology and the increasing understanding of cancer made the field develop too rapidly evolve the areas of modern medicine.

Many people and animals throughout history have been known to have a history of cancer. From the dawn of time in history, scholars have written about cancer and its own origins. Some of the earliest pieces of evidence for cancer was found in ancient Egypt when people found fossilized bone tumors in the human mummies. These scholars also wrote about these tumors in the ancient manuscripts. The growths in the bone were suggestive of a bone cancer and the bone skull destruction was seen in the cancer of the head and neck.

During the time period of the Renaissance, in the 15th century, scientists were continuing to develop a greater understanding of how the human body was able to grow and develop its own traces of illnesses through the environment. Scientists such as Galileo and Newton had started to use the scientific method that was beginning to be used to study diseases. Autopsies began to be led to have an understanding of the circulation of blood throughout the heart and the body. These autopsies were able to relate a patient's illness to pathologic findings after their death. This laid the beginning study of cancer and finding the beginning symptoms. A famous surgeon called John Hunter saw this information and suggested the idea that cancer might be cured by surgery. He described that they might be able to operate on cancer at one point and that one point could be taken out of the body in order to help them survive.

In the 19th century, the birth of scientific oncology was created with the use of the modern microscope with the study of diseased tissue cells. Scientists began to find the paths of cellular pathology that was able to provide the scientific basis for the study of cancer. These methods they used were able to aid in the development for cancer surgery. They would remove the body tissues and examine them in order to find a precise diagnosis. The pathologist was also able to then tell the surgeon if the operation had completely removed cancer through the collection of more body cells that would either be found to be infected or healthy.

In these earlier times, they had found the development of cancer and connected them to different theories. While many physicians have remained confused on the true operations of cancer, they were able to find the symptoms and connect theories to treatment options. The first theory was called the humoral theory. A theory that held the belief that the body had four body fluids: blood, black bile, yellow bile, and phlegm. They thought that if there were too much of one of these fluids, then the disease would start to occur. The second theory was called the lymph theory that was surrounded by the belief that the formation of cancer was caused by another body fluid called lymph. Life was thought to have consisted of the continuous movements of the bodily fluids through the solid parts of the tissues and muscles. Out of all the fluids, they believed that blood and lymph were of the most important. They had another theory that cancer was actually composed of degenerating lymph that varied in density, acidity, and alkalinity. This lymph theory about cancer quickly gained support and acknowledgment. Other surgeons agreed that the tumors grew from the lymph constantly thrown out by the flowing of blood.

The next theory was the Blastema theory that showed that cancer was actually made up of cells and not lymph. The scientist behind this theory also believed that cancer cells actually did not come from normal cells. Instead, they may have come from the budding elements between the normal tissues. He saw that all cells in the body are actually derived from other cells. Another theory is the Chronic Irritation theory that states that cancer is spread like a liquid. This scientist showed that cancer cells metabolize through the spread of other high concentrated malignant cells instead of through another unidentified fluid.

Trauma theory is the theory that states another understanding for cancer. It was thought that trauma would lead to some sort of cancer. This belief was never able to gather a true amount of evidence in order to be seen as even plausible. The Infectious disease theory is a theory concluded by Zacutus Lusitani and Nicholas Tulp. These two doctors showed at the same time that cancer was actually contagious. They made this conclusion through the experiments involving breast cancer in the members of the same household. Later on, they publicized the theory and proposed that patients should be isolated from one another. The first thought was to keep some of the other patients outside of cities and towns in order to stop any chance of spreading the development of cancer. Throughout the 17th and 18th centuries, some people shared this same proposal. The first cancer hospital in France moved away from the city in 1779 since other people feared that cancer would spread throughout the city. Today, research has shown that cancer by itself is not contagious, but it is seen that certain strains of bacteria, viruses, and parasites can actually increase another person's risk of developing a different kind of cancer.

You never know when you are going to hear that someone you know has cancer, but it will probably happen sometime in your life – and it will hit you like thunder.

When you hear someone has cancer, do not just stare and say nothing. Say positive, encouraging words and do not give false hope. People diagnosed with cancer need to feel your support; you do not have to do miracles. Do simple things like making a favorite meal, hold his/her hand, hug him/her, pay the bills, take out the dog, write inspiring notes, watch movies together. Do what you think it would make him/her happy and less worried. Tell him/her that he/she is not alone and that you are there for him/her. Listen and do not focus on the bad things that are happening. Do not cry (when you hear the news it is alright to cry, but later on you definitely should not), the sick person should not feel like he/she needs to take care of you. Tell him/her that he/she is strong and do not let everything you have said to fly in the air. Be there.

When someone has cancer, everybody in his/her life is affected - the whole family, friends, coworkers, etc. The person begins to appear so vulnerable, and you have to be very careful when talking to him/her. Cancer represents abnormal growth of cells. More than 100 types of it are known. Most common types are breast cancer, lung cancer, lymphoma, skin cancer, prostate cancer, blood cancer (leukemia), etc. Cancer is mostly treated with chemotherapy, surgery, and radiation. It is not always successful, but nowadays cancer is far more treatable than it was years ago. It is not an easy job to take care of someone who has cancer. It is a 24-hour job and demanding. Usually, someone related to the patient is their caregiver. It is

[35]

not just about comforting someone. It includes doctor's appointments, chemotherapy, drugs and many other things that appear easy at first glance. You might think that doing groceries, buying drugs, driving the kids, washing the dishes, vacuuming, and all the other everyday activities will be easy. Unfortunately, the caregiver will be overstressed and have the hardest job. Sometimes, even the closest relatives will be tired of caring. It is normal. A person is not a machine that can work all the time. Even the caregiver needs some time off. If you are a caregiver, you should ask for more help. Let other people help your loved one (diagnosed with cancer) and let them help you. It is normal to seek help, at least for house chores. You should not feel guilty when you feel tired of everything. You are a person that has feeling and needs, and you need healthy meals, enough sleep and fresh air (getting out of the car to shop does not count). Do your best.

If you are diagnosed with cancer, do not lose hope. Yes, many will tell you not to lose hope and to be positive. The truth is that it is the best way to cope with anything. Allow yourself to laugh and to do fun stuff. Never miss doctor's appointments or chemotherapy. Do not forget to take medications and do not let the cancer win this battle easily. At first, you will be terrified, and you will refuse to believe what you have heard. It is normal to feel overwhelmed, take your time to process the information. Next step is to get educated. Ask your doctor whatever you want. It is your right to ask and to seek answers. Learn about the type of cancer you have, in what stage you are, is it operable, is it curable, what the treatments are, what side-effects do come along, etc. You are allowed to ask for a second opinion, too. Doctors make mistakes sometimes, but you should be ready to hear it again if it turns out that the diagnosis was correct. If there is a cancer center near where you live, go to get more information. Tell your friends and family. It is always better to share what bothers you. You will cope easier with your disease if you get some help and support from your loved ones. If you think that you will protect your family by not telling them, you are wrong. They will be more upset if you do not tell them. Everybody will be on the same page and try to do their best to help you. It is too much information to handle on your own. You might think that you are good on your own, that you are strong and independent. You are a human being with emotions, fears, and desires. You could use some help, do not be stubborn. Join the support group and talk with the people who have already experienced things that you are about to experience. You will be prepared and less scared when you know the deal. If there are no cancer support groups where you live, join them on social networks. In the world we live today, you can practically do everything online. Read other people's experiences and collect information. You should not be alone in this. During the treatment, do not back down. It will be hard, and it will not be nice. You need to fight, and you need to believe that you will succeed. You need to move your boundaries to the next level, to believe in miracles and healing. Pray if you believe (and if you have not before). Allow yourself to cry and to feel any emotion. You do not have to be strong all the time, and you are only human. Do not forget that you need to continue living. A little bit differently, but you are not dead. It is not easy to say, but life does go on. You just see it from a new perspective. Do not miss the things you love to do because of cancer. Do things you always wanted to do, call that one person that you love but you are both too proud to call. Do not do it because you think you are going to die (you will one day, but that is not the point). You will feel a lot better when you do these things. Do not pretend that everything is normal, again – do not forget your medications or doctor's appointments, and enjoy life. You will discover so many beautiful things you have not seen

[37]

before. There will be times that you want to give up. That is normal too. But do not let anything break your spirit and your faith. Accept that the world is not fair all the time. Accept that we only live once, too. Surround yourself with positive people and positive thoughts.

Chapter 10: Surgery

Surgery is the branch of medicine that deals with working in the body in order to help it heal. It is used to deal with the physical works of the body structure to eliminate any forms of a disease or to work with the tissue samples in order to diagnose the person with a certain illness.

Surgery is an operation performed by a doctor/doctors and a medical team. What does the doctor do? The doctor tries to fix something that is wrong in human's body. He/she is called a surgeon. Surgeon can also take something out, replace something, insert something in, etc. In most cases, a surgeon is an expert in one area for example heart or bones. No surgeon is a surgeon for everything. It is not that a doctor cannot be that great, there are just too many details in human anatomy and they need to be grouped in certain areas (abdomen, thorax, head, etc). General surgery is a surgical area which covers organs in the abdominal cavity. It includes contents like stomach, pancreas, liver, esophagus, colon, small bowel, gallbladder (together with bile ducts), etc. General surgery can also involve trauma, hernias, breasts, thyroid glands, skin, etc.

General surgeons first learn to operate on organs in abdominal cavity and then sub-specialize in some of the following branches:

Trauma surgery

Trauma surgeons are considered the most cold-headed people. They need to focus and react fast in crises. They are general surgeons that need to be prepared to deal with any emergency including extreme bleeding, thoracotomy, cricothyroidotomy, laparotomy, infections, stab wounds, etc. There is no time to spare, trauma surgeons need to be super fast and think quickly. They cope with situations that involve a lot of adrenalin and blood. They play 'time' game, where they have to do certain thing in a small amount of time and the time is their worst enemy. If the time is up, they lose their game and they lose the patient. They need to be extremely brave and not to panic (or show panic) and to make fast decisions. Usually, people need to train for years to become trauma surgeons, not just because of the techniques but also to learn how to deal with stressful situations and how to cope with everything that they see and to learn that it is impossible to save everyone. We can say that they are in the first line of defense and that their work is one of the hardest ones. Their skills sometimes decide whether the patient is going to live or die. There are millions of factors that are involved in trauma surgery, but doctor's skills are certainly one of the most important ones.

Pediatric surgery

There is a reason why there are very few pediatric surgeons in hospitals. It is one of the hardest fields in medicine, because it not only about cutting something or fixing someone's organs – it is about saving someone's child. A pediatric surgeon does not have one patient- that one patient comes with his/her parents and other people involved that are worried about their loved child. Child is never alone and it is one of the hardest things to deal with. You take your thoughts home and you always think about those who you managed to save - and the ones you have not saved. Pediatric surgeon takes care of minors – fetuses (neonatal surgery which is a pediatric subspecialty), infants, little children and adolescents (up until they are 18 years old). Pediatric surgeon improves the quality of young people's lives. Pediatric surgery became popular in the late 19th century. It started as an idea to fix birth defects. Surgeons began to develop new methods and to use new techniques. The rate of birth defect began to decrease over time and more healthy babies were born. Of course, even today babies can be born with defects but it is much more rare condition that it was in the past. There are 2 subspecialties (one we have mentioned earlier) – fetal surgery and neonatal surgery. Therefore, there are many more experts in this field and many more babies saved even before they are born. Other general surgeons have to train during their education to work with pediatric surgeons. For example, cardiothoracic surgeons, neurosurgeons, trauma surgeons, oncologists, etc. They all need to be ready to operate on a child (or give an opinion) together with pediatric surgeons. Common conditions that they cope with are genetic malformations, conjoined twins separations, tumors, hernias, cleft lip, cleft palate, abdominal and thoracic deformities, brain deformities, etc.

Surgical oncology

This is one of the surgical areas that treats cancer patients. Being a surgical oncologist is a very stressful profession, but it is also very important. Surgical oncologist has to operate on tumors and try to get them out of some organ before it spreads. Time is very important as well as regular checkups. Tumors spread very fast and they need to be treated properly. The surgeon tries to take out as many tumors as he/she can, but sometimes there are too many or they are inoperable. If the tumor had gone in several organs, it is much harder to get rid of it (and sometimes surgeons do not notice all of them or they spread to quickly few days after the surgery).

Cardiothoracic surgery

Cardiothoracic surgery treats organs inside the thoracic cavity: heart, lungs and great blood vessels. In some countries cardiac surgery is separated from thoracic surgery and involves only heart and great vessels of the heart (aorta, superior and inferior vena cava, pulmonary arteries and pulmonary veins).

[41]

Residency for cardiothoracic surgeon takes about 5 do 15 years to be fully trained. It is consisted of three parts: cardio, thoracic and vascular surgery. Later, they can sub-specialize in pediatrics and other fields of medicine. This field of general surgery is also filled up with adrenalin (literally and figuratively) and cardiothoracic surgeons must have still hands and cold head to cope with heart failures and other life-threatening situations that patient can be in. Today, medicine has become much easier for people who have shaky hands and want to become (cardiothoracic) surgeons. The procedures (or a part of them) are performed by a robot. The robot is assisting the surgery and it is a machine which is controlled by the surgeon himself/herself. The robot makes an incision enough big for the surgery to be performed. There are no big scars later and the holes do not need to be big for the surgeons hands to fit in – the robot represents surgeon's hand and performs with much more preciseness. Robot has much smaller 'hands' to perform.

Organ transplantation surgery

Organ transplantation means moving one person's organ to another human body in order to replace recipient's damaged, absent or sick organ. This procedure is very complicated (because of all nerves and blood vessels that need to be reconnected) and it is done by the most qualified surgeons. Organ transplantation does not necessarily mean that some part of the body is transferred to another organism. Sometimes organs (but mostly tissues) are transplanted in the same body. In some cases, like severe injuries, burned skin, etc. surgeons take a piece of skin from some healthy part of the body and transplant it to burned area. These organs or tissues are called autografts. In cases when there are different people involved (the donor and the recipient), organs or tissues that are transplanted are call allografts. Almost everything in the body can be transplanted. Most common organs that are transplanted are kidneys. The following organs and tissues are liver, lungs, heart, intestines, eyes (cornea), bones, muscles, nerves, blood vessels, skin, etc.

When donating, donor can be 'circulatory' dead (when the heart has stopped working), brain dead or alive (when donating one kidney or part of the liver). In most cases, the donor is brain dead but his vital organs are alive. Organs from the donor that is 'circulatory dead' can be restored after he/she has been gone for up to one day (24 hours long). Tissues can be preserved and kept in special conditions, unlike the organs. Except cornea, the tissues can be stored for about half decade or more popular to say – they can be 'banked' (most common expression for keeping semen).

It might sound simple, but many people and governments are against organ transplantation. Some people believe that it is not ethical or that it is a sin to do such things. Another things that is extremely hard to do for a physician is to ask the family of the deceased person to donate the organs. Organs are extremely hard to get and many people who are mourning refuse to sign to consent. Some governments try to raise awareness about organ donation by making laws. Some of laws propose that organs will be donated (if for example the donor is brain dead and his organs are in good shape) unless the family asks differently. But, there are some problems with establishing laws – it is believed that organ trafficking will be much more present and more people will be at danger.

Organ transplantation surgeries are not performed on daily bases because they are extremely complicated to perform. They are challenging and demanding. They can last for hours and after all the effort – organ can still be rejected by recipient's body. Sometimes, the immune system does not support the organ despite the right surgery protocol.

People do not get organ donor cards in most cases because they are afraid that they can be misused. They are partially right. But also, people are not aware how much they can help by donating an organ (organs are useless anyway when people die). Some religions even forbid blood transfusion (blood can be considered as a liquid organ).

People decide what they want to do with their bodies and nobody has the right to tell them otherwise. The only thing that we can do is to raise awareness and to put accent on how important organ donating is. It can save many lives, make them longer and better. It should not be a forced deed. Unlike in China, about 95% of the donor organs are used from the executed prisoners. New technologies try do produce artificial organs that will serve as real ones. New discoveries will definitely change the face of medicine and open new opportunities for organ donations and transplantations.

Vascular surgery

Vascular surgery is another surgical subspecialty. It treats vascular diseases by performing non- or minimally invasive surgeries. The most common procedure is catheter procedure or blood vessels reconstruction. Vascular surgeon takes care of all vascular system except the great heart vessels and brain vessels (cardiothoracic and neurosurgery). Vascular surgery takes care of arteries (for example carotid arteries, iliac arteries, femoral arteries, etc.) and veins, mostly varicose veins. It can also deal with vascular transplantations (tissue).

Neurosurgery

Neurosurgery is much more than watching episodes of Grey's Anatomy and McDreamy operating on inoperable cases (although that would be great). As you know, brain is the least familiar organ in a human body and the trickiest one. Nobody knows all about it and neurosurgical operations are the most dangerous ones (especially when it comes to brain tumors). Also, neurosurgery does not only deal with the brain itself, but it also includes the spinal cord and peripheral nerves (usually treated together with trauma surgeon). Interesting fact is that anesthesia is not used during the 'awake' brain surgery. The patient is awake and the neurosurgeon performs the surgery. This is very important because the surgeon works with different parts of the brain which involve important features like talking, hearing, vision, memory, etc. The surgeon can know whether he/she is invading certain area while operating. Operation is very stressful for the patient, starting from the drill sound (nobody is thrilled by the fact that someone is making a hole in their skull) and the fact that the patient's brain is exposed. Neurosurgeons treat many conditions like head trauma, traumatic injuries, psychiatric disorders, epilepsy, tumors of the brain, spinal cord and even peripheral nerves, hydrocephalus, meningitis, intracranial hemorrhage, brain stimulation surgeries, etc. Like any other field in medicine it is very stressful but also extremely important. Nothing about neurosurgery is safe and the surgeon cannot know whether the surgery went well until the patient wakes up. Some patients die on the table and some end up in a coma (brain dead). Neurosurgery meets with a lot of opportunities for organ donations. Neurosurgeon deals not only with loses and unsuccessful operations due to aggressive tumors or bleeding, but also with convincing the families to sign the consent for organ donating. Being a neurosurgeon is very hard and demanding job.

Not every surgery requires panic and asking for extra blood. Some surgeries are very simple and painless. For example, taking the tooth out is considered a very easy surgery. On the other hand, some surgeries can be extremely hard and full of risks. Some people even die on the table. Easy surgeries can turn in complicated ones. The surgeon never knows how the surgery is going to end. Surgery can be very complicated, demanding and unpredictable. Surgery is performed in a very clean place, doctors and nurses scrub in (wash their hands, forearms and nails and wear special clothes –scrubs). Everybody in the operating room need to wear scrubs, hats, clean shoes, masks and gloves. The place is called an operating room (OR). Some hospitals have multiple operating rooms. Operating rooms are very clean and nurses keep it clean before, during and after the surgery. It has to be clean non-stop. It has to be germ-free and full of necessary equipment. Nobody but medical staff and the patient cannot enter the operating room. Patients are put to sleep with using anesthetic (the use of anesthetic is called anesthesia). They cannot feel the pain during surgery. Anesthetic can be rubbed on the skin, given by gas for a patient to take a deep breath or given by injection. It blocks the pain receptors and provides painless procedures. Before modern anesthesia people (doctors) used alcohol, cocaine and some other psychoactive substances. Joseph Lister first developed modern anesthesia.

Surgery used to be one horrible and terrifying procedure. It is nothing like that anymore. Of course, many people have fear of going under the surgeon's scalpel, but it will probably happen to every human being once in a lifetime. It is not fun as going to some roller coaster, but is also not as terrible as it seems. People should think that surgery is their way out, the best thing that can happen to them. You have probably read somewhere that a patient had a 'life changing surgery'- most of the surgeries are like that. Surgeries are invented to cure, not to harm anybody. There are risks, but much more benefits. Surgery used to be dangerous, painful, and something like bad horror movie. It was the last chance and many people died on the table. It was stressful and unfortunately very few people lived when surgery was first invented.

[46]

Since human beings were first able to create sets of tools and develop ideas of medicine, surgical techniques began to develop. Each time they practiced, they learned another part of the body and how it is able to function. Once they reached the times of the industrial revolution, the surgeons were not capable of truly overcoming the three main principle obstacles that continued to plague the medical profession. These three things are bleeding, pain, and infection. While advances in this scientific field worked to transform the ways of surgery, they wanted to stop surgery from being a risk and have it become a more reliable source of treatment for people to follow.

The first surgical techniques were created to treat different cases of injury and trauma. They would first work to amputate limbs and drain out the open wounds. Once they let out enough blood, they cauterized the wound. On Asian tribes, they used a mixer of a saltpeter and sulfur to place on the wounds and lit it with a match in order to cauterize the wound. The people in Dakota were able to use the quill of a feather attached to another animal bladder to take out any material. During the Stone Age, they discovered the use of needles that were used to cut long the skin. The tribes in India and South America were able to develop their own method for sealing up minor injuries. They would put termites and other insects on the wound and counted on them to eat around the edges of the wound. After, they would twist the neck and leave their heads attached to the skin as if they were staples. Overall, the oldest operation known to existence was called trepanation. This technique came from the Greek people who would drill a hole into the skull to expose the infected area. By doing this, they released the pressure inside the skull and were able to treat other health problems. These early techniques were taken fully into account each time as they were created to improve the cultures and the health of the people around them. Each one developed a new form of knowledge that could be used for information later on.

Being a surgeon means that you are a special kind of person. Not everyone can be a surgeon. It is not an easy job at all. Many people become surgeons because of the adrenaline they feel when they open the body up when they cut the flesh and fix anything that is wrong in the body. Saving someone's life is the biggest pleasure and rush anyone can feel. That feeling cannot be compared to any other feeling in this wo rld. You have to take the risk. You have to be both mentally and physically strong to conquer anything that happens to you. When your pager beeps in the middle of the night, you never know who you will see in the operating room. Sometimes, the things you have learned in school do not work. Not every patient can be saved the same way; not everything works the same on the same people. Sometimes, you have to forget about textbooks, about everything you have learned and try something new because when you do all that you already know (and it does not work) – there is nothing else left to do.

Conclusion

In this series of information involving the influence of viruses and antibiotics, it can be seen how the world of medicine began to develop. People were truly interested in helping each other and getting each other to better health. From the kindness of nurses to the research of scientists, everyone played their part in the medical field and how hospitals themselves came into the modern age.

Starting with the thought of how people experimented with different techniques, each thought built upon another. While people today may not think about how surgery first began, it did start the foundation that began what we have today.

Medicine is not just about wearing scrubs and a white coat. It is so much more. Healing someone is the greatest thing in the world. Helping someone is the most beautiful thing in the world. Being a doctor is not just a job, it is a lifestyle. If you choose to join it, you have to know that from the minute you enter college, your life will never be the same. Your habits change, as well as your daily routine, friends, obligations, you will never look at the world in the same way as you did before. By being a medical student, nurse, doctor or any other medical worker, you devote your life to humanity. Your patient is your concern. His/her life is in your hands. You have to put yourself out there and do your best to help somebody.

It does not matter are you a neurosurgeon, a scrub nurse, a pediatrician, radiologist, etc. You are one of the most useful human beings in the world. Because of you, people get better. People heal and go back to their daily routines. Your daily routine is part of making the world less painful. You are probably not aware of your importance. When you go to bed, picture all the people that you saved or you were a part of their healing. Feels great, right? Nothing in this world can replace the feeling and the satisfaction of being a medical worker. It is not always rainbows and butterflies, to be honest, it is almost never rainbows and butterflies. But then it happens – you see that patient that was in your office a month ago, buying balloons in the store for his/her child's party. And the patient is standing on his/her feet, smiling. You see that lady that you saved six months ago, walking with her husband in the city. You see that kid jumping in front of his/her school and playing with her/his buddies, and you see that man who was a kidney recipient drinking his favorite juice in the cafeteria. All those people are alive because of you. It does not matter whether you did their x-ray scan, draw some blood from their veins or operated on their brain. You did something. You saved that person. You made this world   greater. They all are better because you were the part of their healing process. You managed to do something useful. How does it feel to see that kid you operated on? That is rainbows and butterflies. That is the dream of every medical professional. It makes you forget all the year of pain, struggles, and tears. It makes you forget sleepless nights, failed exams, madness, and rage. It makes you full of joy and dopamine. It makes you feel like you did something right. That is worth living and studying for. That is worth everything.

Thank you for purchasing this book and taking the time to read through it. Please leave a review saying what you enjoyed or what else you would have liked to have seen. The purpose of this book is to give you some new information, and to help you get some new perspective.

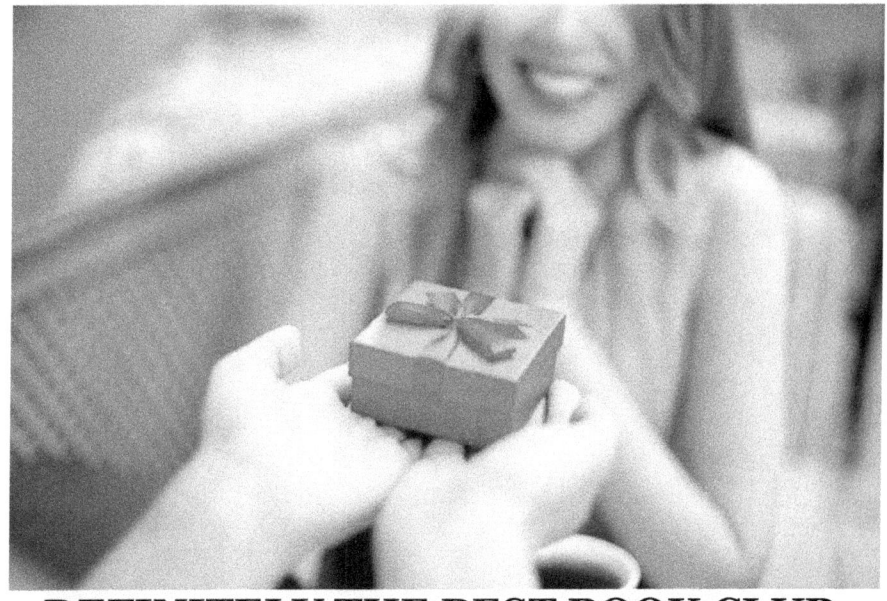
[51]